TOWN & HOME

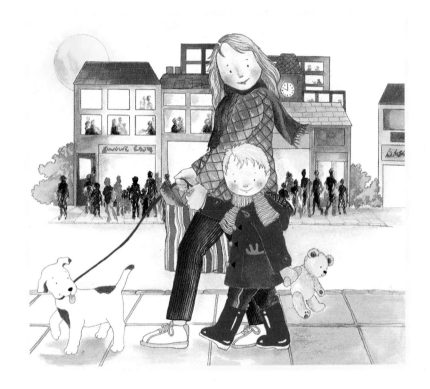

Written by Linda Baillie
Illustrated by Pip Shuckburgh

MALLARD
PRESS

To Sarah, Katie and William

This edition published by Mallard Press,
an imprint of BDD Promotional Book Company, Inc.,
666 Fifth Avenue, New York, New York 10103.
Mallard Press and its accompanying design and logo
are trademarks of BDD Promotional Book Company, Inc.
Originally published in the UK by Blackie and Son Ltd.
as IN THE TOWN and IN THE HOME.

The publisher, distributor and copyright holder wish
to point out that the information in this book is for
reference and discussion only, and should not be
used as a substitute for parental advice and attention.

TOWN

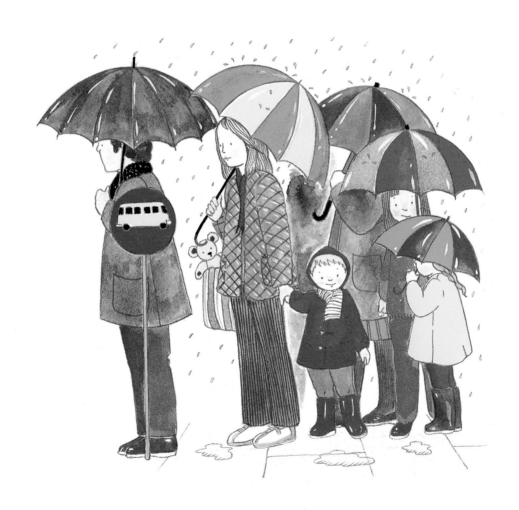

Jack and Teddy are going shopping with Mom.
Jack loves going into town. It is always very busy,
with lots of things to see and do.

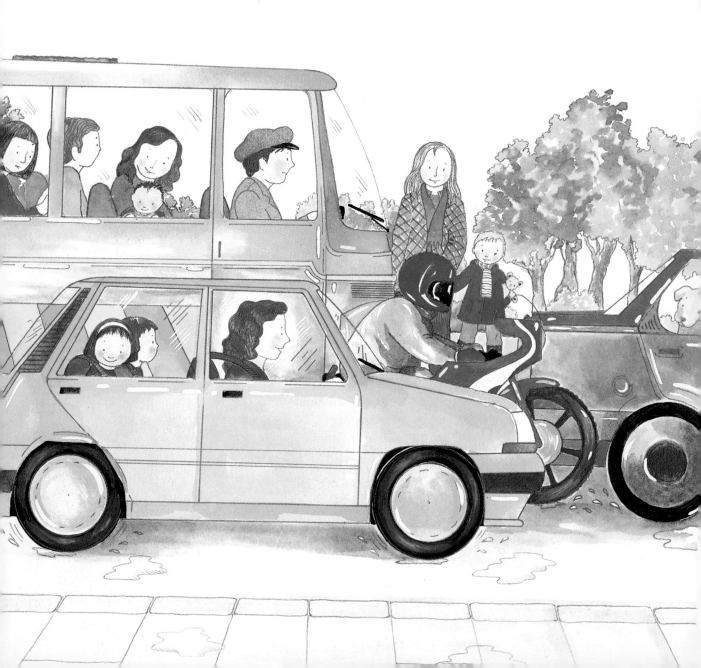

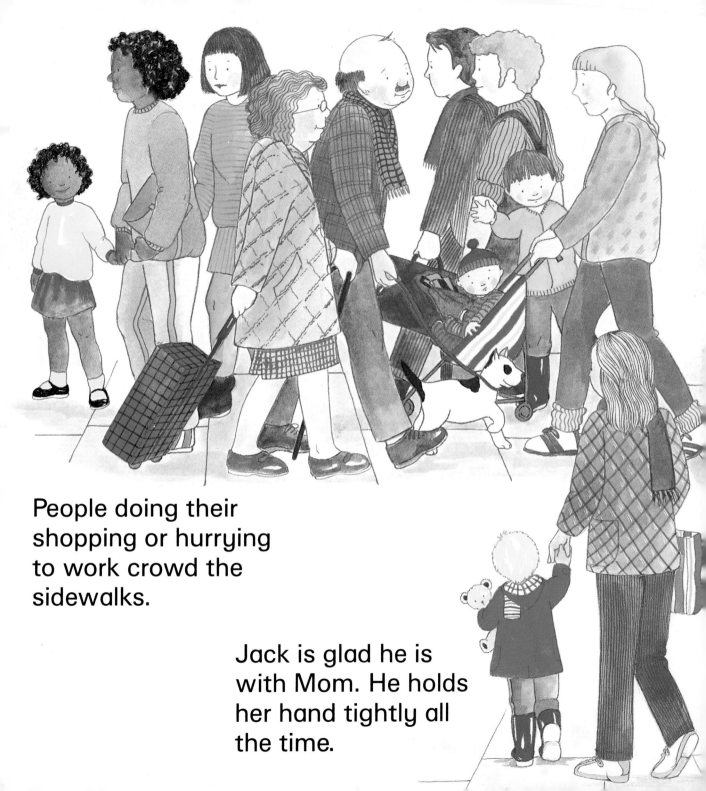

People doing their shopping or hurrying to work crowd the sidewalks.

Jack is glad he is with Mom. He holds her hand tightly all the time.

Sometimes Jack goes to town in the car. Here it is, parked outside his house. Jack knows the color of his mom's car so he can find it in the street. Can you see what color it is?

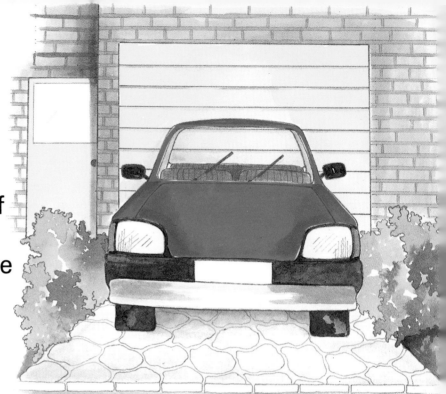

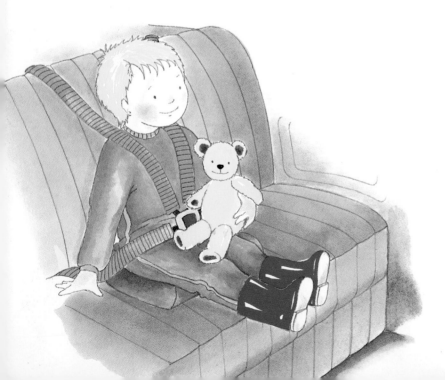

Jack climbs onto his booster seat in the back. His mom straps him into his seat belt.

Jack keeps very quiet while Mom is driving. Sometimes he listens to a story or songs on the radio.

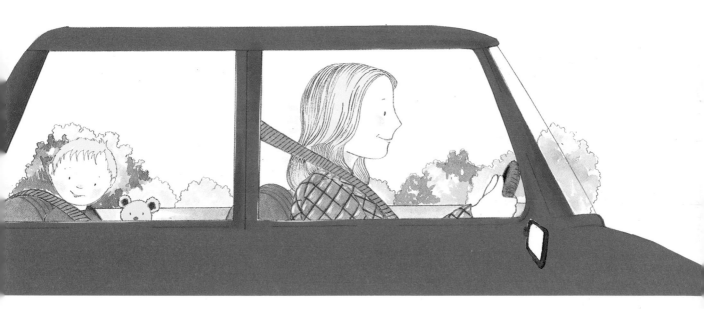

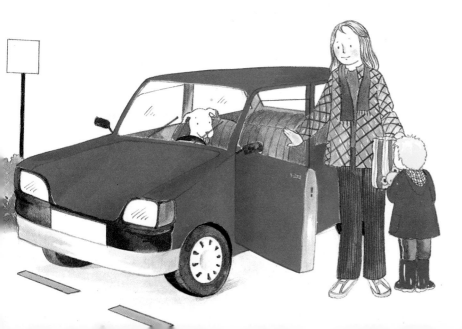

Jack sits still while Mom parks the car and opens the door. If they bring their dog and they aren't going to be long, they leave him in the car with a window slightly open.

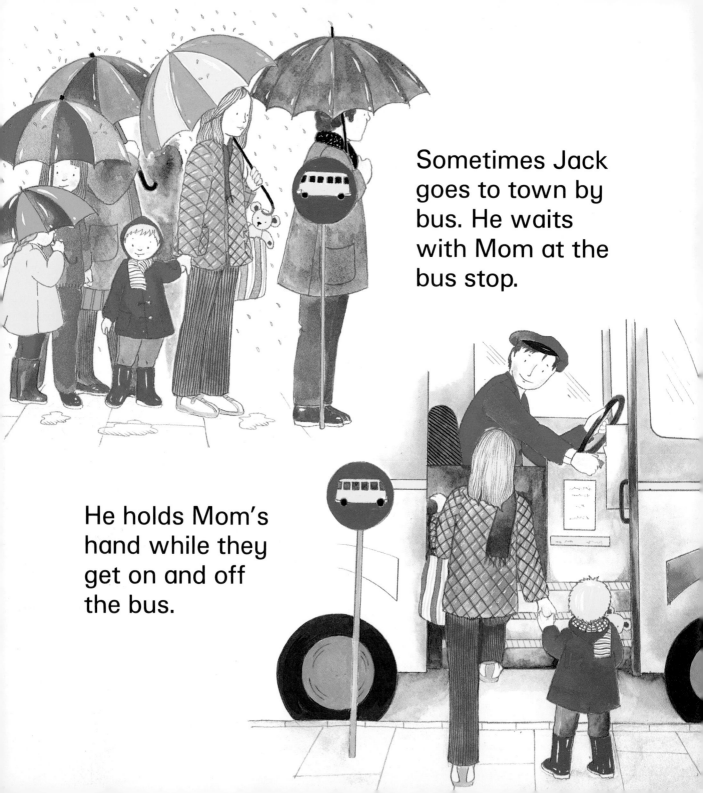

Sometimes Jack goes to town by bus. He waits with Mom at the bus stop.

He holds Mom's hand while they get on and off the bus.

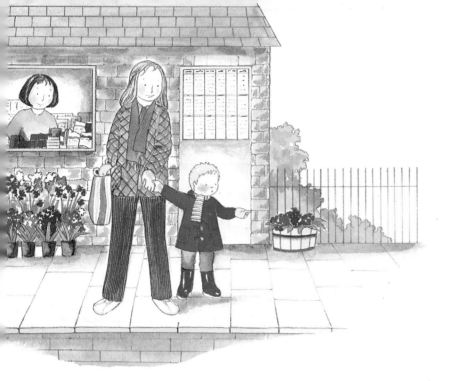

Sometimes they take the train. Mom buys their tickets and they wait on the platform together. Don't get too near the edge, Jack!

Mom helps Jack to get on and off the train.

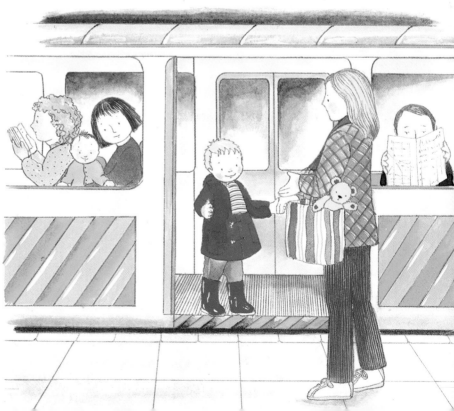

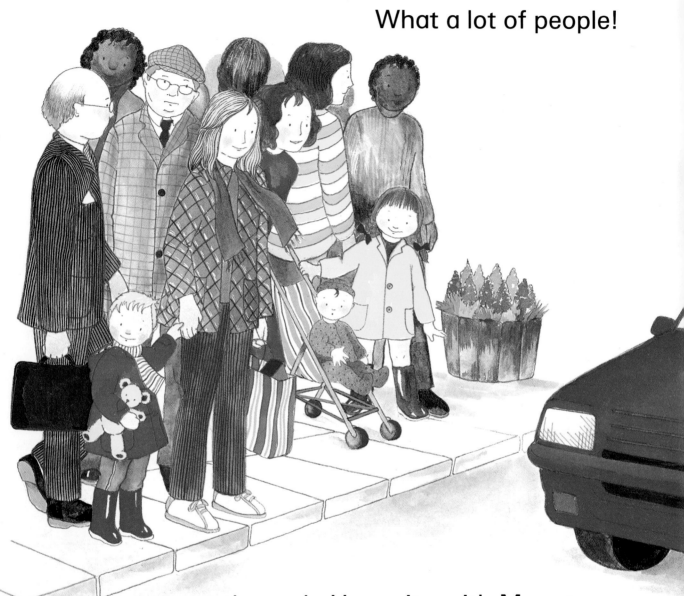

What a lot of people!

Jack stops at the curb. He waits with Mom to cross the street. They find a place with no parked cars so they can see. They look all around for traffic and they listen carefully, too.

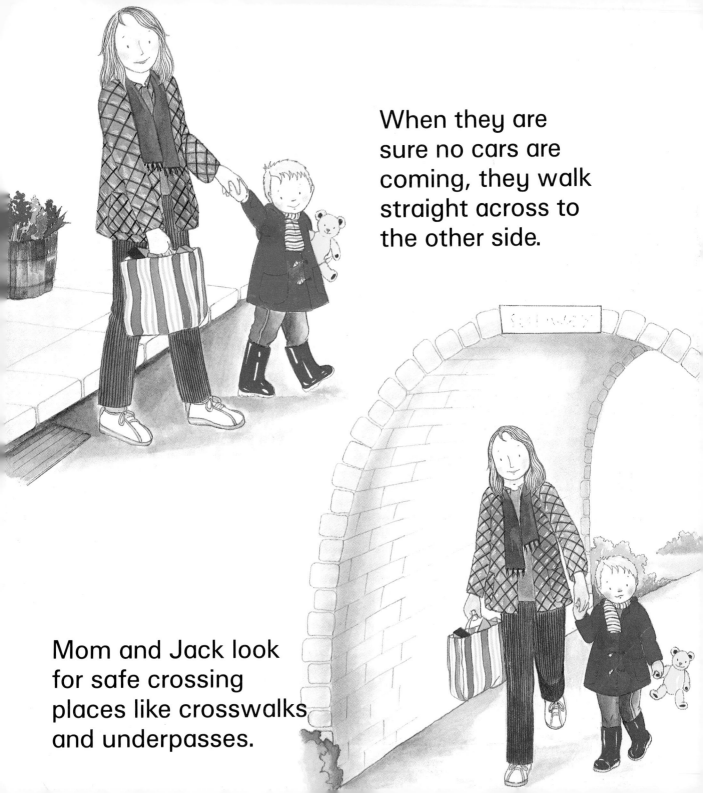

When they are sure no cars are coming, they walk straight across to the other side.

Mom and Jack look for safe crossing places like crosswalks and underpasses.

Policemen and crossing guards will help Jack cross the street. If he gets lost he can tell them his name and address and they will help him. Salespeople will help him, too, but Jack does not speak to anyone else he does not know.

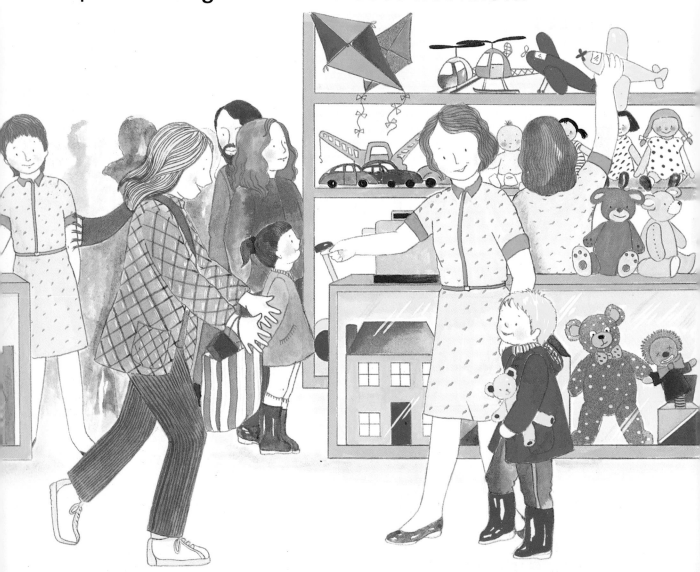

When there are a lot of people around, Jack always stays very close to his mom.

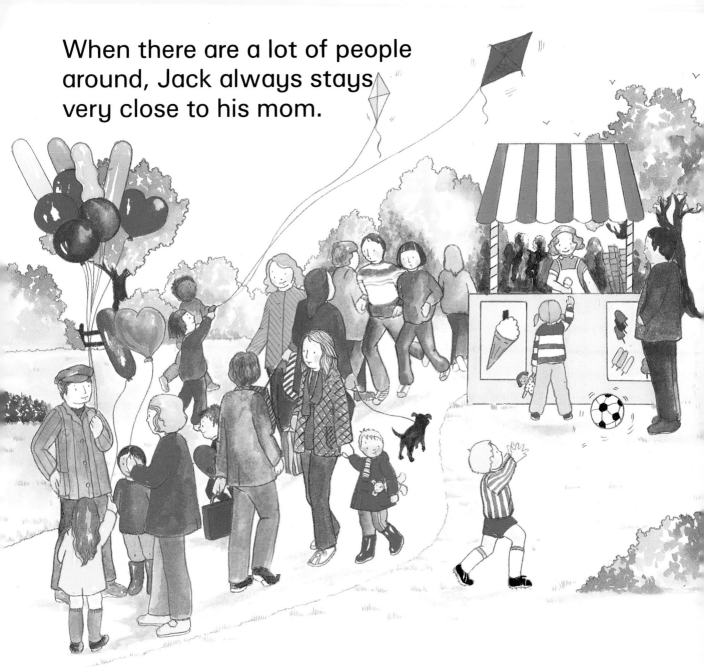

He remembers what she is wearing so he can find her in a crowd. Can you see what Jack's mom is wearing today?

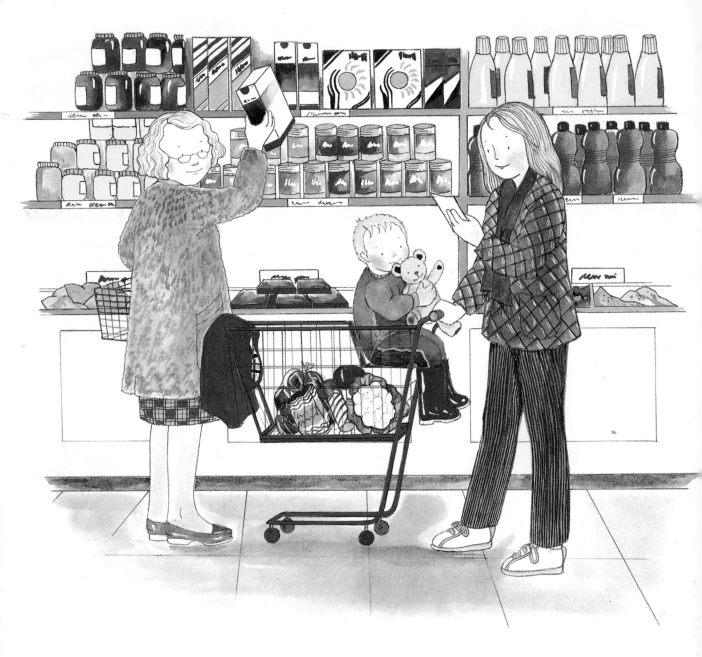

A supermarket is an exciting place because it sells all sorts of things. Jack sits in the shopping cart and helps his mom choose what to buy.

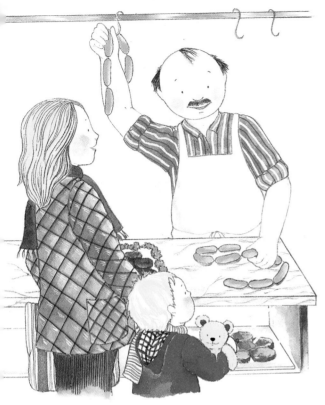

Mom goes to the butcher's counter for some meat and to the bakery section for some bread.

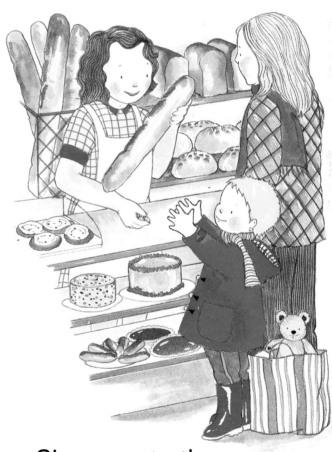

She goes to the produce section for some vegetables and fruit.

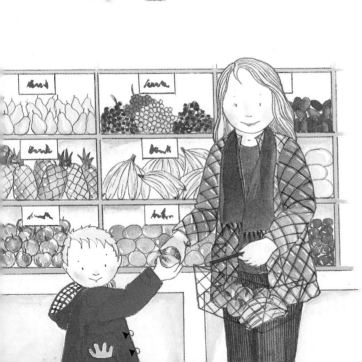

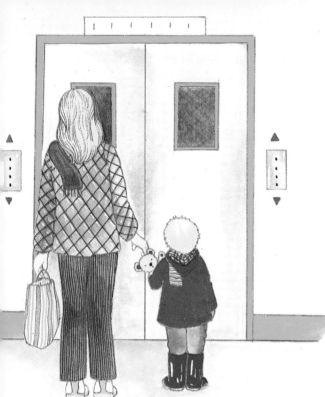

Jack likes
department stores,
too, because they
have escalators
and elevators
to take him up
and down.

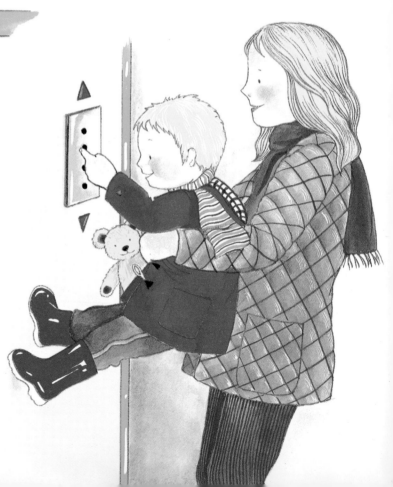

Mom lets Jack
press the elevator
button. "Going
up!" he says.

Jack holds his mom's hand when he is on an escalator.

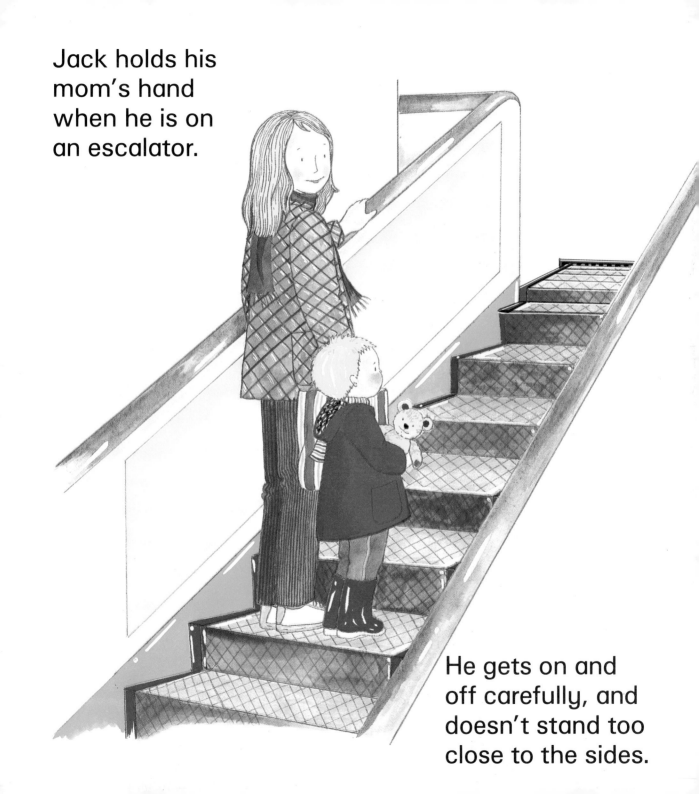

He gets on and off carefully, and doesn't stand too close to the sides.

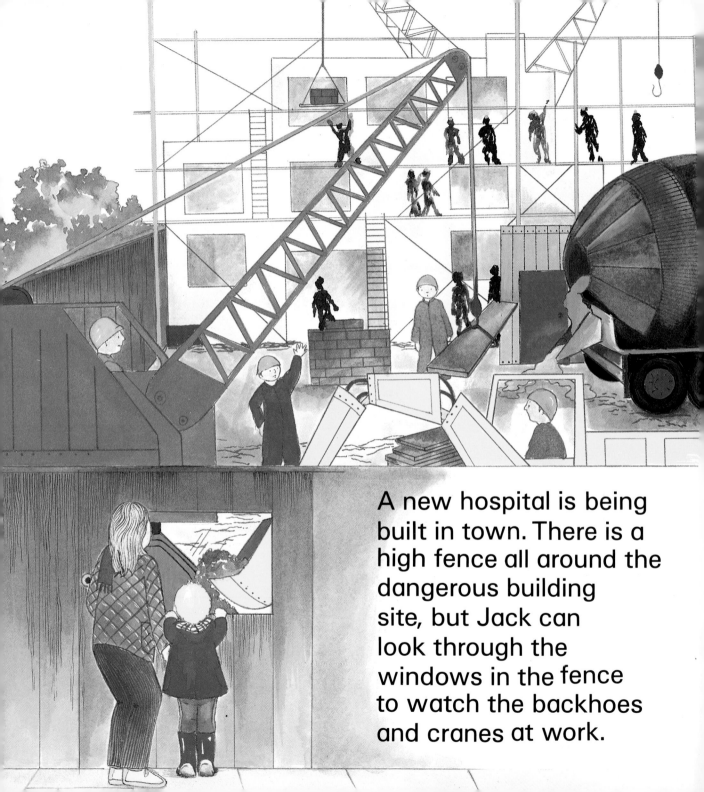

A new hospital is being built in town. There is a high fence all around the dangerous building site, but Jack can look through the windows in the fence to watch the backhoes and cranes at work.

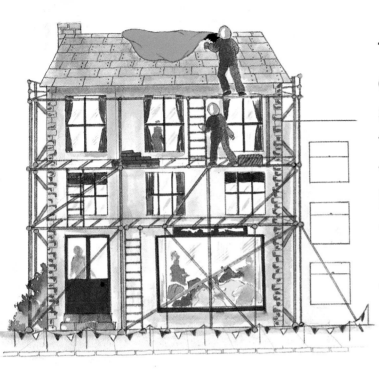

This store is covered in scaffolding so that the builders can fix the roof. Jack loves to watch all the busy workmen, but he never goes too close.

Jack likes to see the bulldozers best of all. They push the dirt around.

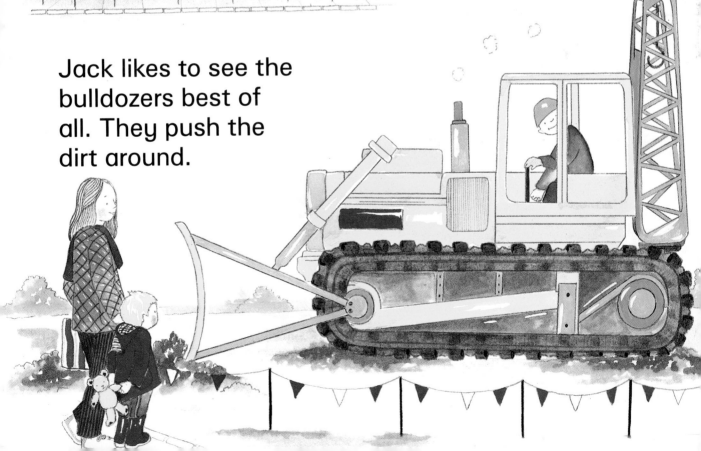

Look, there's a fire engine with flashing lights!

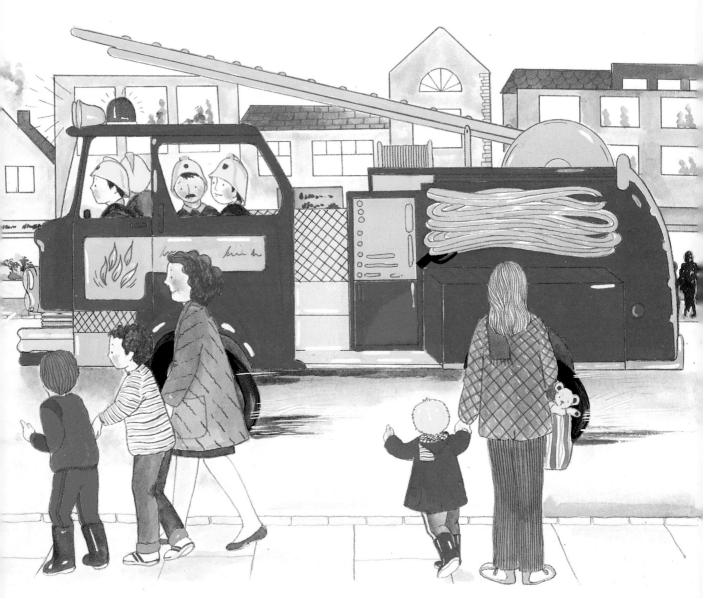

There is always a lot happening in the town where Jack lives. Sometimes he sees a police car or an ambulance go rushing by.

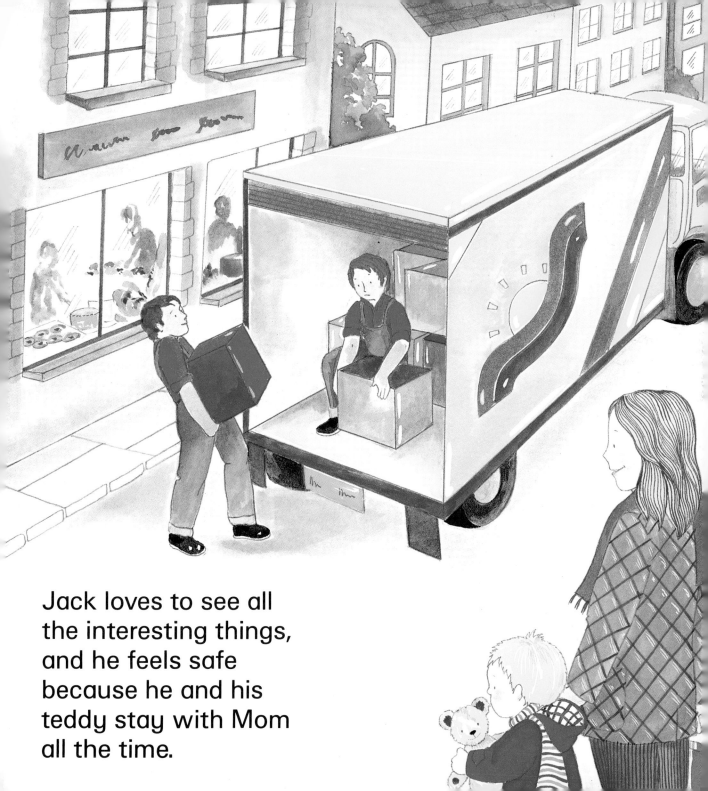

Jack loves to see all
the interesting things,
and he feels safe
because he and his
teddy stay with Mom
all the time.

HOME

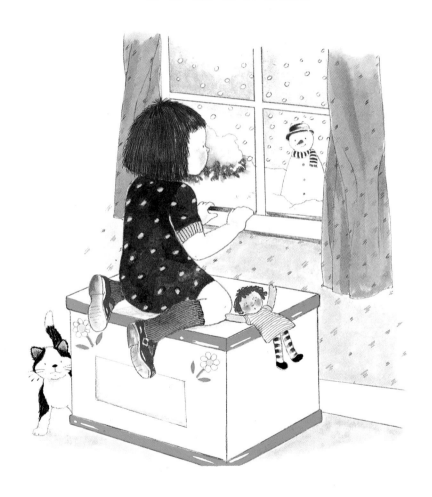

This is Rosie's house.

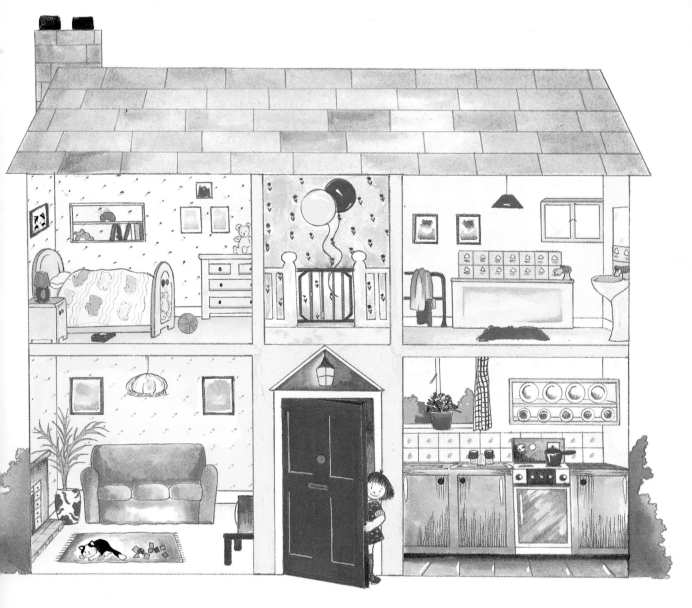

There is a kitchen to cook in, a living room to sit in, a bathroom to wash in, and bedrooms to sleep in.

Rosie knows all the
best places to play
in her house.

She knows
the places
where she
must be
extra
careful.

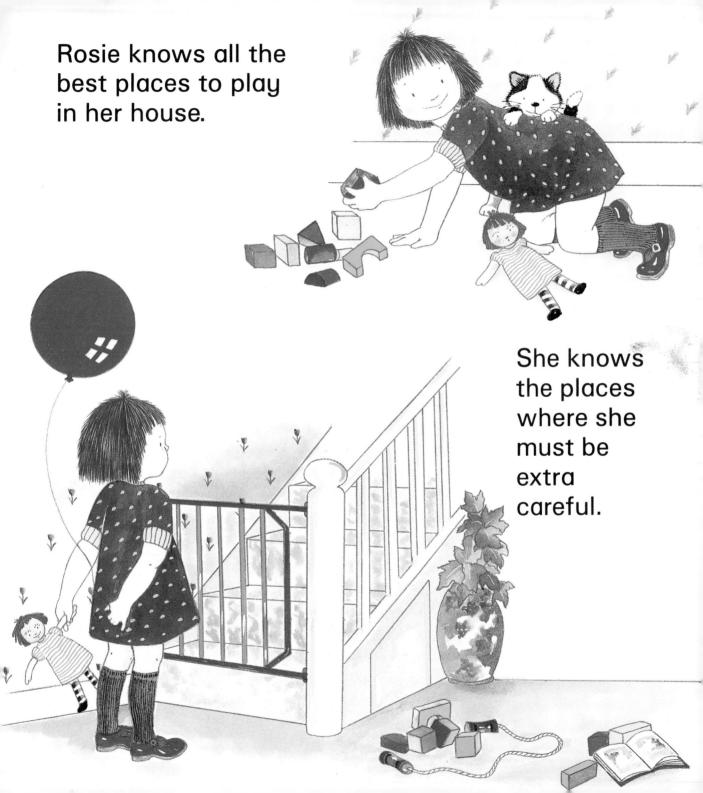

Every room has a door and some windows.

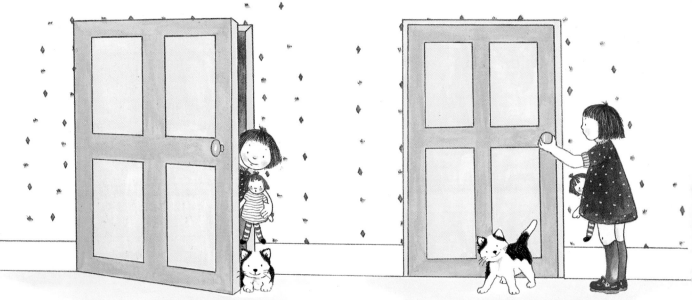

Look, there's Rosie opening her bedroom door.
She closes it very quietly. Be careful of your
fingers, Rosie!

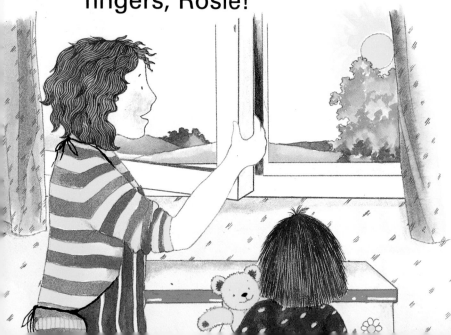

On sunny days
Mom opens the
windows. Rosie
knows she
shouldn't lean
out of them. Do
you know why?

The stairs have a gate at the top and a gate at the bottom.

"Can you help me go down the stairs, Mom?" says Rosie.

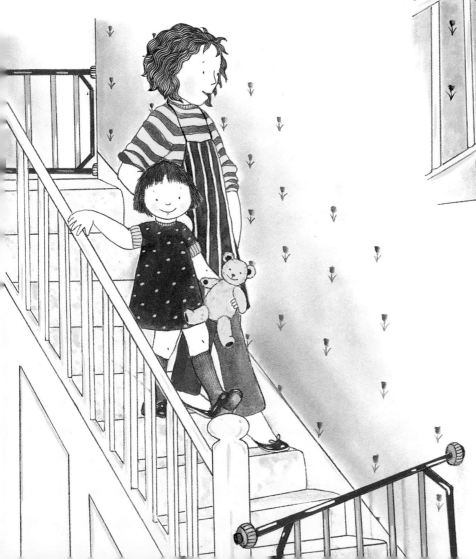

"I'll hold on to the bannister," says Rosie. "One step, two steps, three steps . . . look, it's easy!"

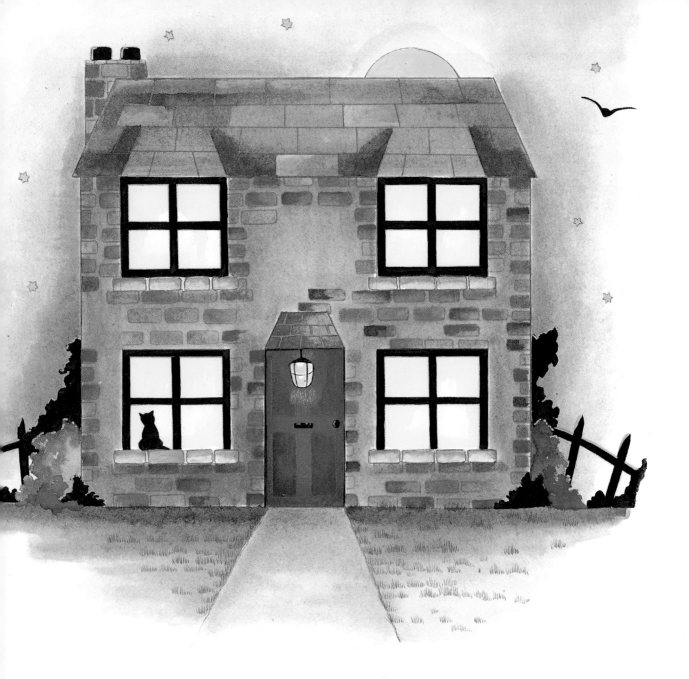

When it is dark outside Mom and Dad turn on the lights. There are switches in every room.

Electricity makes the lights and the television work.

Rosie knows that she must not touch the knobs or switches. If she wants something turned on or off, she asks a grown-up to help her.

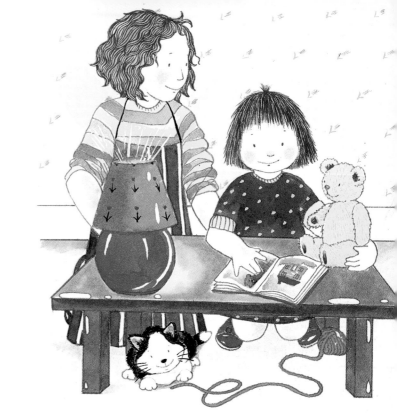

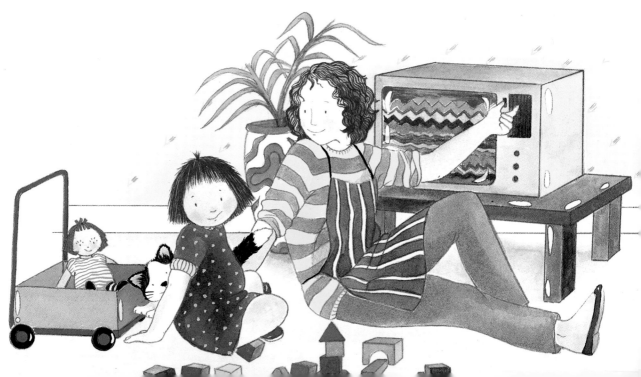

Watching television is fun. But Rosie knows not to touch the wires or the plug.

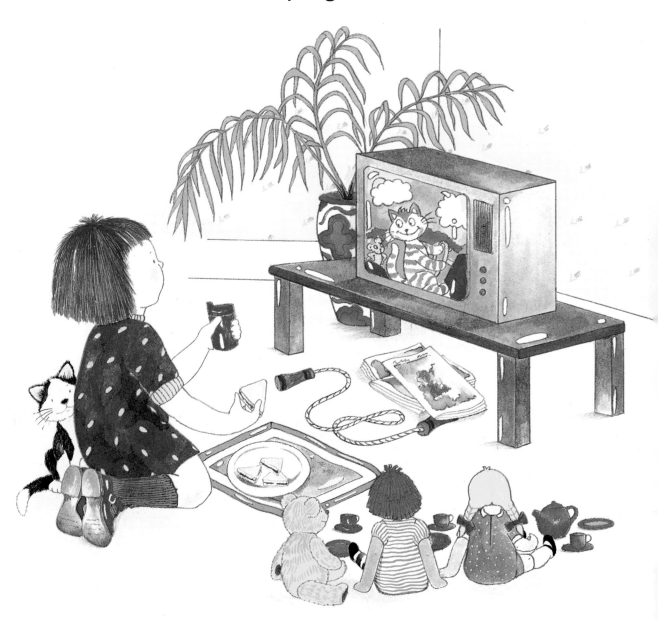

Look, Rosie's toys are watching, too!

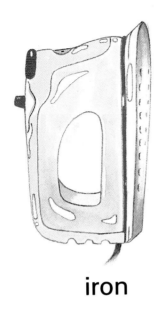

iron

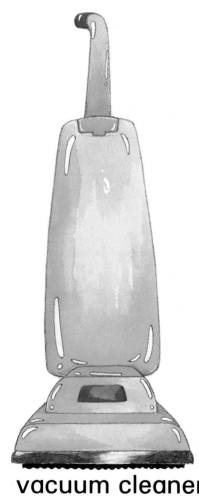

vacuum cleaner

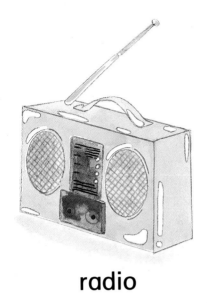

radio

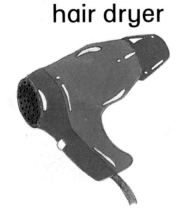

hair dryer

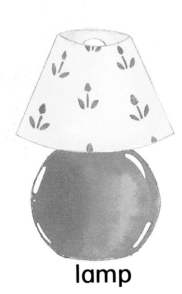

lamp

Electricity runs all these things in Rosie's house.
What things does electricity run in your house?

When it is cold outside Rosie plays inside. When the heat is on she feels snug and warm.

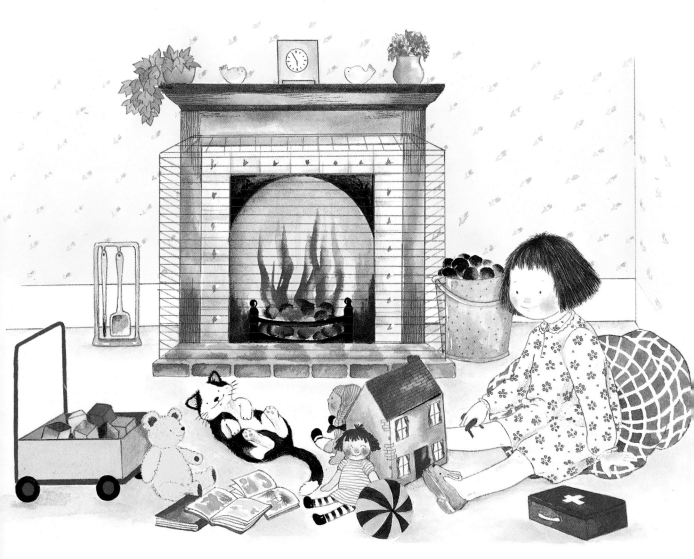

Some fireplaces burn logs or coal, and some run on electricity or gas. Fire screens are put in front of them to keep them safe, but don't go too close!

Rosie has some radiators around her house. Do you have them, too?
Radiators can get quite hot, so watch your fingers!

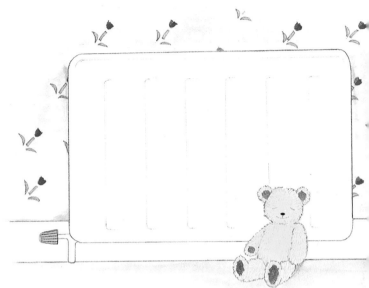

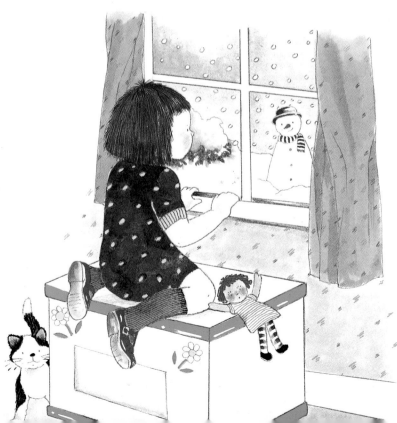

The fires and radiators make the house cozy and warm, even on the coldest day.

Rosie likes to help in the kitchen. "You can help with the dishes," says Mom. "We'll make sure that the water is not too hot, and that there are no dishes that could cut you or anything that might get broken."

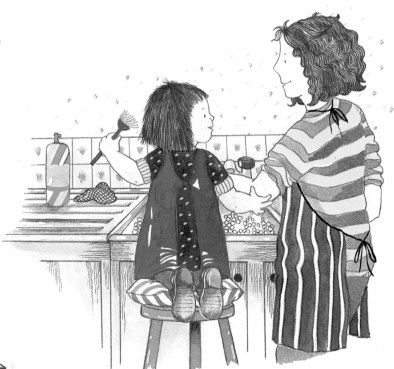

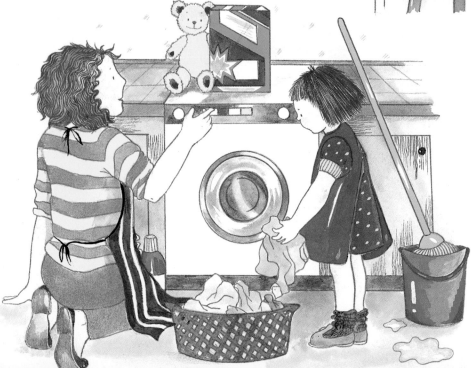

Rosie helps load the washing machine. In goes all the dirty laundry. Mom puts in some detergent and turns on the machine.

Rosie can make gingerbread men. They go into the oven to bake. The oven gets very hot, so Rosie doesn't touch it. Mom takes the cookies out when they are ready. ''Mmm, they smell good,'' says Rosie.

Rosie has her own cup to drink from. It has a special lid on it, so she can drink from it easily without spilling anything.

Rosie does her painting on the kitchen table.

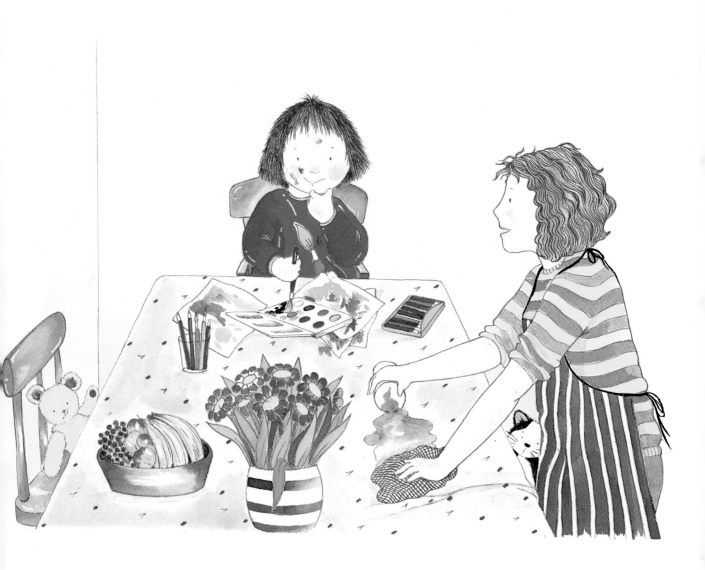

Oops, the paint has spilled! Now it needs to be cleaned up.

There is a cleaning closet full of mops and brushes, buckets and dust cloths. There are bottles of liquid for cleaning floors, walls, and windows.

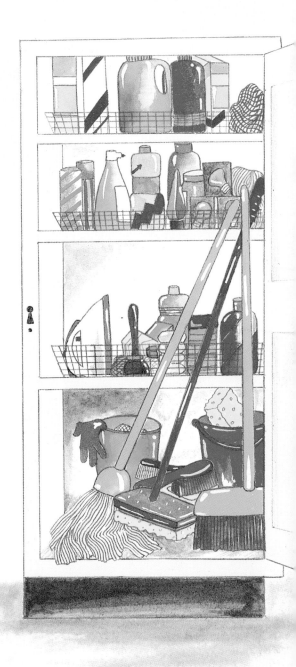

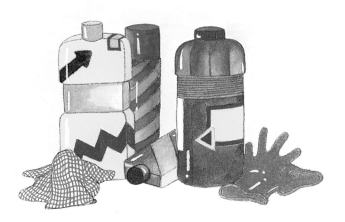

Most of the bottles have special tops and only grown-ups can open them, because the liquid inside can make you sick. That's why all the cleaning supplies must be kept away from children.

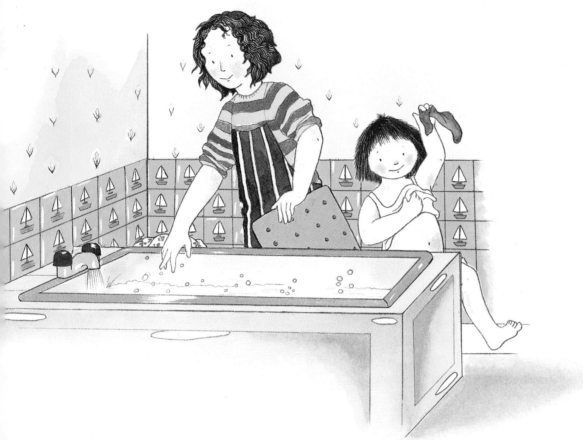

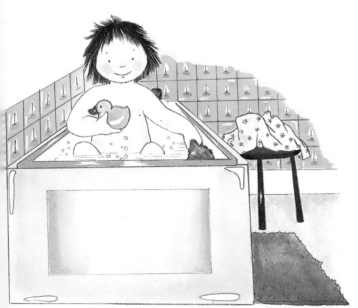

"It's time for a bath," says Mom. She runs the water — not too hot and not too cold. It's just right for Rosie! She sits on a rubber mat to stop her from slipping.

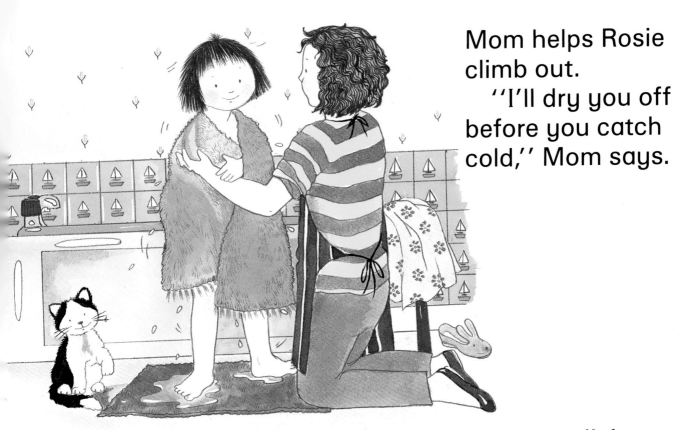

Mom helps Rosie climb out.

"I'll dry you off before you catch cold," Mom says.

In the bathroom there is a cabinet with medicine inside it. Only grown-ups are allowed to open it.

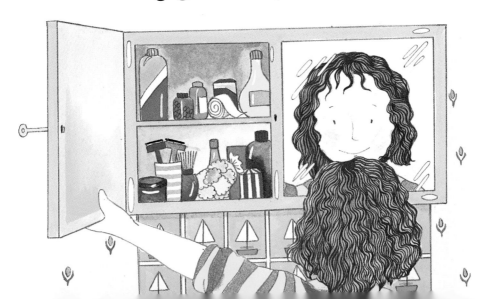

Rosie is clean and sleepy when she hops into her bed at the end of the day. She loves her cozy bedroom with all her toys around her. The curtains shut out the dark night outside.

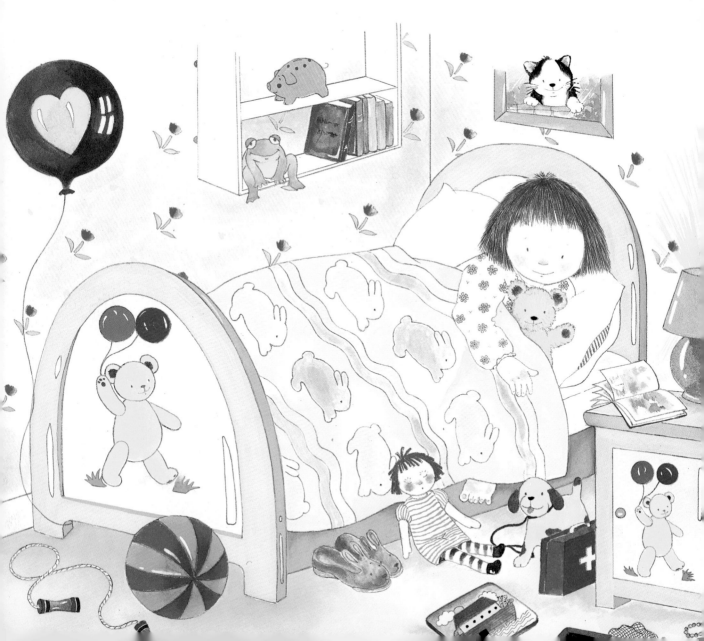

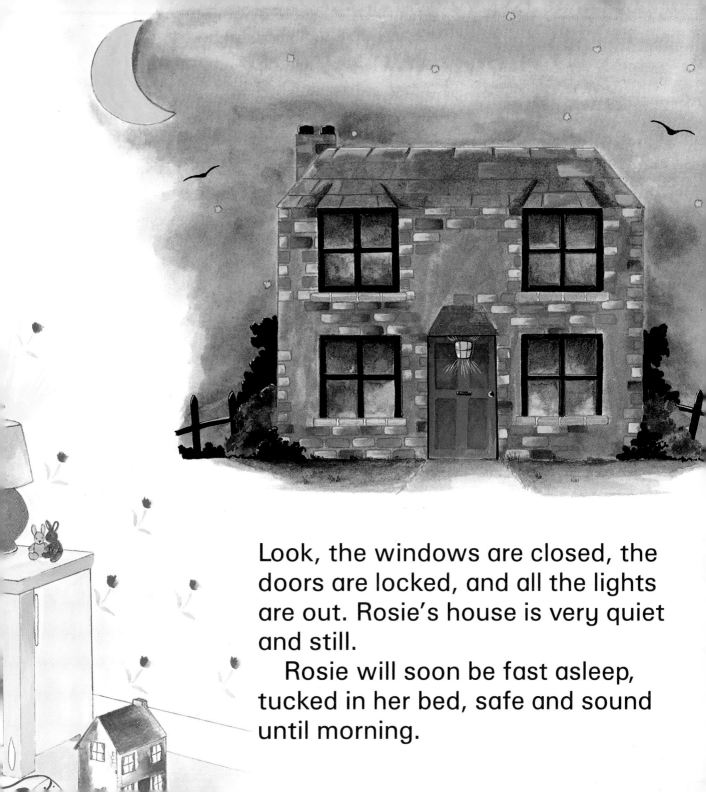

Look, the windows are closed, the doors are locked, and all the lights are out. Rosie's house is very quiet and still.

Rosie will soon be fast asleep, tucked in her bed, safe and sound until morning.